YOUR KNOWLEDGE HAS VALUE

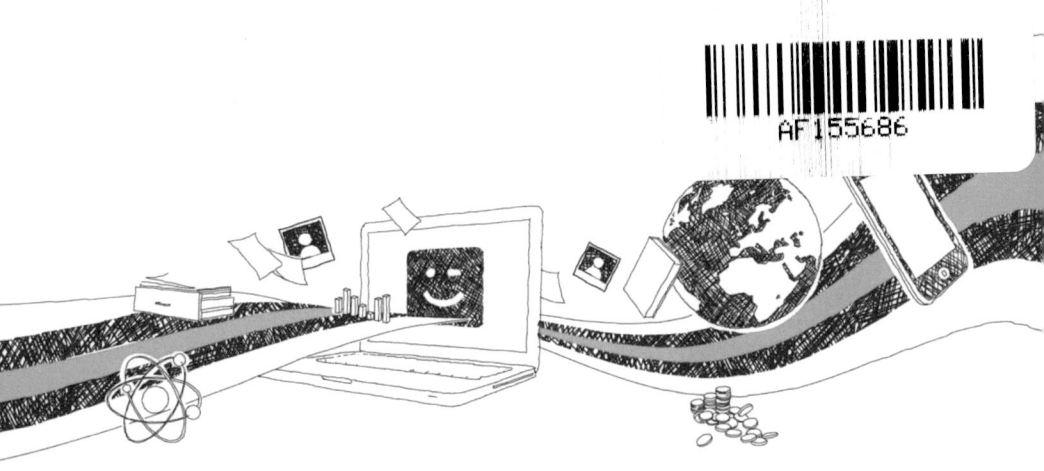

- We will publish your bachelor's and master's thesis, essays and papers

- Your own eBook and book - sold worldwide in all relevant shops

- Earn money with each sale

Upload your text at www.GRIN.com and publish for free

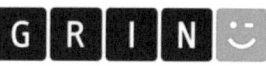

Bibliographic information published by the German National Library:

The German National Library lists this publication in the National Bibliography; detailed bibliographic data are available on the Internet at http://dnb.dnb.de .

Imprint:

Copyright © 2016 GRIN Verlag, Open Publishing GmbH
Print and binding: Books on Demand GmbH, Norderstedt Germany
ISBN: 9783668381322

This book at GRIN:

http://www.grin.com/en/e-book/351379/young-people-s-sexual-reproductive-health-in-uganda

Jenkins Tanga

Young people's sexual reproductive health in Uganda

GRIN Publishing

GRIN - Your knowledge has value

Since its foundation in 1998, GRIN has specialized in publishing academic texts by students, college teachers and other academics as e-book and printed book. The website www.grin.com is an ideal platform for presenting term papers, final papers, scientific essays, dissertations and specialist books.

Visit us on the internet:

http://www.grin.com/

http://www.facebook.com/grincom

http://www.twitter.com/grin_com

YOUNG PEOPLE'S SEXUAL REPRODUCTIVE HEALTH IN UGANDA

In the next decades, Uganda is expected to have the highest population growth in the world (Worldwatch, 2016), as already observed with a population increase of 10.7 million people between the two national censuses of 2012 and 2014 (UBOS & UNFPA, 2014). As of January 2016, the population of Uganda was estimated to have increased by 3.58% (countrymeters, 2016). Uganda possesses a large rural population, which has a high unmet need for contraception. Indeed, Uganda has high Total Fertility Rates (TFRs), reaching 6.2 in 2011 according to UDHS 2011, which puts pressure on the reproductive health services. Although since 2000 Uganda has been implementing a Sector Wide Approach (SWAp) to health sector coordination and support (WHO, Country Operation Strategy at a Glance, 2014), its population still needs to resolve urgent Sexual and Reproductive Health (SRH) issues.

This report will look at the SRH of young people who are defined as those between the age of 15-24; this age bracket also covers the crucial adolescent age bracket of 15-19 years. This report begins with an introduction which gives a background on the state of Uganda and the sprouting of its health system. These two factors have a direct and an imminent impact on the state of SRH, its policy, achievements and challenges. This report will further describe the main data sources and its collection. It will then focus on four areas of young people's SRH notably contraception and fertility, maternal health, abortion and HIV/AIDS. Each field consists of trends and patterns, programmes, policies and challenges. Finally, the conclusion will describe the future of SRH in Uganda.

Content

Introduction

Uganda gained its independence on the 9th of October 1962 and is in the preliminary stages of its demographic transition. With a large rural population and TFR averaging between 6 and 7 lifetime births per woman, only about 18% of women between the age 15 and 49 use effective contraception (Haub & Gribble , 2011). Like many other developing countries, Uganda has gone through a series of civil conflicts that have had negative impacts on young people's SRH. For example, the Lord's Resistance Army conflict in Northern Uganda challenged Adolescents' SRH (ASRH) as there was massive violations manifested by atrocities like rape, induced abortion, unwanted pregnancy and interferences with SRH data collection. Uganda's health system is based on user charges and cost sharing, where hospitals have to charge for treatment thereby making it difficult for adolescents to obtain adequate SRH. Thus, Ugandan women teenagers have more births compared to older women, with approximately 15% of births occurring to mothers below the age of 20 as opposed to 12% occurring to mothers above 35 years (MOH, n.d). These factors highlight the unmet need for contraception among the adolescents in Uganda.

Main Data Sources:

The main data sources were the Uganda Demographic and Health Surveys (UDHS), Uganda AIDS Indicator Surveys (UAIS) and censuses. The DHS generally collects information on health and population, including on SRH, in developing countries. Five UDHS and two UAIS were conducted in Uganda and contain information on ASRH, maternal health, HIV/AIDS, family planning and violence against women. The national DHS was useful for comparative purposes because it used the same sampling methods and data collection instruments. As aforementioned, Uganda is no stranger to civil conflicts, as observed in the Northern and Western regions, which over time affected the national coverage of the surveys, thus leaving national coverage to the 2006 and 2011 surveys. However, this lack of data is also a disadvantage since it makes comparison of data difficult. Additionally, it should be noted that every ten-year census provides additional useful information on a host of issues ranging from fertility to adolescent maternity, though as noted by UBOS (2008), the depth of data when compared with DHS is quite limited. Published qualitative studies that focus on young people's use of SRH services also significantly contributed to the data.

Fertility and Contraception

Generally, the TFR of Uganda has been declining in the past years, yet at a relatively slow pace, as shown in Fig 1. Now ranking fifth, recent data shows that Uganda reduced its TFR to 5.97 in 2014 (indexmundi, 2015)

By the release of Uganda's population report in 2012, Uganda was considered as the country with the world's youngest population, having 78% of its population below 30 years old. The report further revealed that 52% were below 15 years (population Secretariat & UNFPA, 2012). This percentage today, represents a massive young population that the government and social services struggle to deal with.

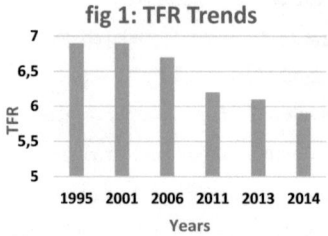

Source: Authors own graph with data from UDHS 2011 and Indexmundi

In addition, in Uganda, high fertility among the young population aged 15-24 years has become a serious public health concern (Nalwadda et al, 2010). As of 2009, approximately 49% of the population was below 15 years old and 20% was between 15 and 24 years old (PRB, 2009). Therefore, the majority of young people in Uganda today face the potential risk of unwanted and unplanned pregnancy. However, similar to TFR, adolescent fertility rate has decreased in the country to 115 births per 1000 women ages (15-19) in 2014 as shown in Fig 2. Despite this steady decline, the rates remain high.

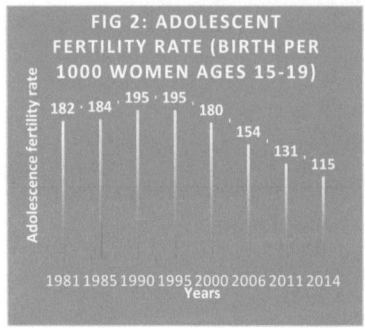

Source: Authors own graph with data from (World Bank, 2016)

One of the major reasons for high TFRs among the youth of Uganda is the early age of first sexual intercourse amongst couples. The first sexual intercourse for women is one year less

4

than their median age of first marriage (17.9 years) whereas that of men is four years less than their median age of first marriage (22.3 years) (UDHS 2011). This warrants increased need for contraceptive use as it exposes young women to the risk of pregnancy (Nalwadda et al 2010). UDHS 2011 shows that 24% of teenagers have either given birth or are pregnant, a slight reduction from the UDHS 2006 that put pregnant teenagers at 25%. These statistics are quite troublesome to policymakers, health specialists and demographers alike. The high percentage of adolescents initiating child bearing at an early age can be linked to the persistently high fertility levels (Rutaremwa, 2013). Ironically, it should be noted that pre-marital sex is highly defamed culturally but this is a disadvantage in its own as it prevents young people from seeking SRH services like contraceptives. In a country with generally low levels of contraceptive use, contraception use is equally low for young people. The UDHS 2011 data shows that only 14% of currently married women aged 15-19 use any form of contraception. Interestingly, although the awareness levels about contraceptive methods are quite high, the usage is significantly low. Nalwadda et al (2011) showed that 98% of population are aware of at least one method of contraception, however, only 10-20% reported using modern contraception apart from condoms. In another study, it was noted that chances of contraception use were higher amongst young women who had given birth before age 15 (Kabagenyi et al 2016), signifying the behavior change which comes in after birth (Rutaremwa, 2013) and the low use of contraception amongst young people. With such high unmet need, lowering the fertility levels turns out to be a formidable challenge.

Policies and Challenges:

Policies aiming to improve SRH of young people have been put in place by the government. Notably, policies date as far back as 1999 with National Minimum Healthcare Package that entailed young people SRH (MOH, 1999), Adolescent Health Policy Guidelines and Service Standards (MOH, 2001). Ensuing policies aimed at influencing the future demographic trends and patterns to improve the adolescent health. To do so, policies encourage fertility reduction, literacy improvements, SRH expansion, increased use of contraceptives as well as of trained health personnel involved in delivery (Neema et al, 2004). To address ASRH issues, Uganda's first comprehensive National Adolescent Health Policy was approved in 2004 (Rosen, 2005) and Health Sector Strategic and Investment Plan were initiated in 2010 (MOH, 2010). Furthermore, in 2006 Uganda signed the Maputo plan of action which aims to ensure that the continent achieves universal access to comprehensive SRH by 2015 through improvement of SRH of young people (AUC, 2006) A number of polices have been implemented to deal with the SRH but the young population has been reluctant when it comes to seeking SRH services. Indeed, qualitative studies revealed that young people's usage of SRH services in Uganda is hampered by not only techincal issues but also by socio-cultural issues that create barriers. A study by Kisaakye (2013) noted that nearly a third of providers would not supply contraceptives to individuals younger than 18, unmarried, still in school, and those without children, even though the policy guidelines of Uganda do not have such requirements. Similarly, in Kabarole district, another study highlighted the same reason of lack of privacy and confidentiality for lack of SRH services among the young people (Kipp et al, 2007). Thus, misconceptions and negative attitudes towards SRH are the biggest challenges and barriers that need to be addressed to improve the SRH of young people in Uganda. Policies should not only address contraceptives provision but should also encompass the broader aspect of young people SRH.

Maternal health

Although some progress has been made in Uganda in regards to maternal health, MMR remains significantly high at 343 deaths (World Bank 2015). At least six women survive with chronic and debilitating ill health for every maternal death in Uganda (WHO, 2011). In Uganda, women marry at a very young age as over half are married before the age of 18 (MoFPED, 1996). This purports that women aged 20-24 years old give birth before the age of 18 with 33% giving birth before the age of 18 and 6.6% before 15 (UDHS 2011). This therefore creates a problem for young people's SRH as pregnancy among adolescents is linked to high morbidity and mortality for both mother and child. Though adolescent pregnancy has been steadily declining in Uganda (41% in 1995, 31% in 2000, 25% 2006), it is still high (Atuyambe, 2008). Hence it represents a considerable challenge to health service providers. Antenatal care (ANC) can address some of these hindrances by reducing the number of future complications both during and after delivery. However, most adolescents either book very late for the second phase of ANC or do not attend at all (Atuyambe, 2008), which can make child bearing life-threatening for young people. Adolescent pregnancy in Uganda is asssociated with increased risks of adverse pregnancy outcomes and yet unsafe abortion, pregnancy, child birth and obstertric complications such as obstructed labor and severe bleeding lead to most maternal deaths. Of salient concern in Uganda is obstetric fistula that occurs during labor and birth when the infants head is too big to be pushed out but it has already entered the maternal pelvis. This usually happens when the expectant mother's pelvis is underdeveloped, the infant is too big or is mispositioned. Because young people in Uganda initiate sexual intercourse early in their lives, they are highly prone to such risks.

Policies and challenge

With the adoption of liberal family planning policies like the National Adolescent Health Policy, Health Sector Strategic Plan of 2000, Reproductive Health Strategy, and the National Obstetric Fistula Strategy of 2012, the government has effectively tried to influence a behavioural change amongst the youth. Moreover, the recently concluded initiative of accelerating the reduction of maternal, neonatal mortality and morbidity in Uganda (2007-2015) showed that the government has identified ways of improving family planning, improving on Emergency obstetric care (Emoc), increasing access to antenatal care and trained personnel with the needs of the youth.

However challenges remain especially since adolescents are reluctant when it comes to seeking SRH services and they cannot be solely blamed for this. Indeed, a Ugandan study showed that adolescent mothers faced increased community stigmatization and violence that fostered poorer health seeking behaviour for both them and their children (Atuyambe, 2008). They are deprived of SRH services as they lack support from their spouses and family which in-turn neccesitates a lack of user fee for hospitals (Nansubuga , 2011), hence inadequate use of SRH services.

Abortion

It should be noted that Uganda lacks abortion data on ASHR, as shown in the DHS pgW-7 that has one question, "Did you have any miscarriages, abortions or stillbirths that ended before 2006?". This question is addressed to the women and not specifcially to young adolescent females.

Unsafe abortions, unplanned births and maternal injury and death are a common occurance in Uganda because of high levels of unintended pregnancies. Dr. Charles Kiggundu in a presentation to the Ministry of Health in February 2014 noted that many women lost their lives due to unsafe abortion. Of the 400,000 aborted cases out of one million unwanted pregnancies every year, 90,000 of them result in severe complications (Musoke, 2014). As different studies use different techinques, measuring the impacts caused by abortion becomes difficult. Because Uganda has no legal abortion services except when saving a life, adolescents are more at risk of unwanted pregnancies, unsafe abortion may follow (Ssengooba et al, 2004). Unintended pregnancies are particularly common amongst adolescents and young people because of premaritial sex, as more than one in three never-married women aged 15-24 have had sex (Hussain, 2013). About 15-23% of female youths aged 15-24 who had ever been pregnant had had an abortion (Ssengooba et al, 2004). Because of the stigma associated with early pregnancy and later abortion in Uganda, youth are more likely to seek unsafe abortion and are reluctant to openly seek SRH services like post-abortion care and counseling that they need.

<u>Polices and Challenges</u>

Striking praise goes to the expressed concern about the morbidity and mortality arising from abortion manifested in the Ugandan Penal Code of 15 June 1950, which makes abortion unlawful (Population Policy data Bank). Indeed, under section 141 "Any person who, with intent to procure the miscarriage of a woman whether she is or is not with child, unlawfully administers to her or causes her to take any poison or other noxious thing or uses any force of any kind, or uses any other means, commits a felony and is liable to imprisonment for fourteen years" and section 143 that makes the supply of drugs or any thing for the facilitation of abortion is illegal with three years of imprisonment (ILO, 2013). However, this does not mean that it is not justified as the law permits its use when saving a life of a pregnant woman under section 224. The loop hole here is that the law does not state the exact circumstances under which abortion is legal, which represents a disadvantage in itself. The government also initiated a Health Policy Strategy of Health Sub-Districts (HSD). The HSD had the objective of improving access to minimum health care package and decentralizing health service delivery to the community level through bottom-up approach with key services such as post-abortion care and Emoc (Ssengooba et al, 2004). Lack of proper and full implementation of health policies greatly affects Uganda (Wallace, 2011).

Moreover, there is limited capacity for health facilities to manage abortion complications despite the latter remaining a major contributor to maternal morbidity and mortality. A study noted that post-abortion care was poorly facilitated as there was shortage of equipments, drugs and supplies, and above all a lack of skilled personnel to handle abortion cases in health facilities (Mbonye, 2000). Treatment of unsafe abortion complications is expensive as the post abortion care on average costs US$ 130 (Hussain, 2013) thus a hinderence to youth seeking these services as it becomes very expensive for them. Regardless of the expensive care, the biggest problem is lack of transparency due to corruption and embezzlement of public funds that delays the initiatives.

HIV/AIDS

Uganda adopted the ABC (Abstain, Be faithful and if you can't, use a Condom) campaign to fight against HIV/AIDS in the late 20th century. With this campaign, it focused on the 'zero grazing' strategy, which targets older men who had disposable income thereby giving them leverage to have multiple coherent sexual partners. The main data sources of information for this are the Uganda AIDS Indicator Survey 2011 (UAIS) and Uganda AIDS reports. These were used to find vital HIV/AIDS statistics with a focus on young population aged 15-24 years. According to the UAIS 2011, in the twelve months leading to the survey, 31% and 32% of unmarried women and men respectively aged 15-24 had had sex, with less than half of both young women and men reporting the use of condom. This shows that youth are more prone to HIV/AIDS due to their risky sexual beahviour. In 2013, Ugandan youth aged 15-24 had a prevalence rate of 4.2% for women and 2.4% for men, a difference that can be attributed to gender-bias in access to education, health services, social protection and information about how to cope with injustice (AVERT, 2015). Because of the rapid roll out of anti-retroviral treatment (ART), the possibility of infants to live through adolescence has been made possible. However, their special needs are not addressed as the existing programs are based on adult care (Birungi, et al., 2008).

Youth in urban areas have an upper hand as compared to those living in rural areas when it comes to HIV knowledge with 49% compared to 35% in urban and rural areas respectively (MOH, 2012). With regard to multiple sexual partners, young men had a higher percentage (10%) as compared to women (3%). Only 24% of women and 31% of men report the use of condom, pointing out that for men, the level of multiple sexual partners changes with age (MOH, 2012). Indeed, as the men age, they start to acquire more disposable income because of their elevated status due to factors like jobs, hence having more sexual partners.

Policies and Challenges

With the government's commitment to fight HIV/AIDS, a number of policies have been set up to tackle this issue. The HIV Sentinel Surveillance System was established in 1989 to provide information on the magnitude and trends of HIV infection in the country as well as to inform strategic planning, monitoring and evaluation (MOH, 2012). However, most of its data is on pregnant women and limited to sentinel clinics. Since then there have been several policies targetting HIV/AIDS, including the National policy for HIV testing and Counselling, National youth policy and school health policy with strategies such as The Uganda National Plan for eMTCT, National SRH/HIV linkages and integration Strategy, National Condom

Strategy 2013-2015, National Comprehensive Condom Programming (CCP), TB-HIV Collaborative Activities Strategic Plan 2013-2015, Leadership Advocacy Strategy on HIV/AIDS, Guidelines for HIV/AIDS Coordination at Decentralized Levels in Uganda, 2013 (Uganda Aids Commission, 2014). The country has also tried to reach out to the youth engaged in adolescent sexual activity through different partnerships with the UNAIDS, WHO, UNICEF, UNFPA and WFP (Uganda Aids Commission, 2015). HIV-related stigma and discrimination is a notable challenge, which affects the reproductive health of those living with HIV. Another challenging factor is that HIV treatment programmes in Uganda are still organised around adult and pediatric care and fail to address the special needs of the youth (Birungi, et al., 2008), simply because most programs consider the youth living with HIV as asexual while ignoring the fact that they have sexual desires too.

Future Sexual Reproductive Health

The focus of this report was on the youth SRH of Uganda, focalizing on four principle themes. Although the government has adopted a number of effective policies in order to alleviate SRH problems, a lot more needs to be done. It has been observed that the data and policies related to the special needs of the youth is lacking as most of the interventions and government studies are centered on the SRH of the general population. Being in its initial stages of a demographic transition, Uganda urgently needs to design policies that specifically target adolescents and the youth.

On a positive note, the free access to mass media has enabled the smooth running of different programs targeting the youth such as 'OBULAMU program' which has helped address youth SRH. Policies like the National Adolescent Health Policy, and National Policy for HIV Counselling and Testing are commendable as they permit adolescents as young as 12 years old to go for HIV testing without parental consent. Similarly, the Uganda National Policy Guidelines and Service Standards for Reproductive Health includes a section specifically addressing ASRH that demonstrates the government's active partipation towards effective youth SRH. As noted by UDHS 1995, education is key since women with secondary education tend to marry later than those without education. Uganda has done a tremendous job in improving primary and secondary education, initiating the provision of 1.5 points to young women joining higher learning institutions whilst integrating SRH into the school curriculums. However, most of the information does not reach many youth as the adults who are responsible for the transmission of this information still disseminate inaccurate information.

Of salient concern is the serious reflection on youth SRH needs as looking through the questionnaires of the various surveys, I noted that there are no direct questions related to SRH for the young population. This therefore leads to the generalization of SRH services while ignoring the specific SRH needs of the youth.

Bibliography

Atuyambe, M. L. (2008). *Adolescent Motherhood in Uganda: Dilemas, Health Seeking Behaviour and Coping Responses.* Stockholm: Kardinska Institutet and Makerere University.

AUC, A. (2006, September 18-22). *Plan of Action on Sexual and Reproductive Health and Rights (Maputo Plan of Action).* Retrieved from Special Session The African Union Conference of Ministers of Health Maputo, Mozambique: https://pages.au.int/sites/default/files/MPoA_0.pdf

AVERT. (2015, May 01). *HIV and AIDS in Uganda.* Retrieved from AVERT: Averting HIV and AIDS: www.avert.org/professionals/hiv-around-world/sub-saharan-africa/uganda

Birungi, H., Mugisha, J. F., Nyombi, J., Obare, F., Evelia, H., & Nyinkavu, H. (2008). *Sexual and Reproductive Health needs of adolescents perinatally infected with HIV in Uganda.* FRONTIERS program.

countrymeters. (2016). *Uganda Population.* Retrieved from countrymeters: http://countrymeters.info/en/Uganda

Haub, C., & Gribble , J. (2011). The World at 7 Billion. *Population Bulletin, 66*(2). Retrieved from http://www.prb.org/pdf11/world-at-7-billion.pdf

Hussain, R. (2013). *Unintended Pregnancy and Abortion in Uganda.* New York: Guttmacher Institute. Retrieved from Guttmacher Institute .

ILO. (2013, 3 19). *NATLEX Uganda.* Retrieved from International Labour Organisation: http://www.ilo.org/dyn/natlex/natlex4.detail?p_lang=en&p_isn=75312&p_country=UGA&p_count=130

indexmundi. (2015, June 30). *Uganda Total Fertility Rate .* Retrieved from index mundi: www.indexmundi.com/Uganda/total_fertility_rate.html

Kabagenyi, A., Habaasa , G., & Rutaremwa, G. (2016). Low Contraceptive Use among Young Females in Uganda: Does birth history and age at birth have an influence? analysis of 2011 Demographic and Health Survey. *Journal of Contraceptive Studies.*

Kipp , W., Chacko, S., Laing, L., & Kabagambe, G. (2007). Adolescent reproductive health in Uganda: issues related to access and quality of care. *Int J Adolesc Med Health, 19*(4), 383-93.

Kisaakye, P. (2013). *Determinants of Unmet Need for Contraception to Space and Limit Births among Various Groups of Currently Married Women in Uganda.* Regional Institute for Population Studies University of Ghana, Legon.

Mbonye, A. (2000). Abortion in Uganda: Magnitude and Implications. *African Journal of Reproductive Health, 4*(2), 104-108. Retrieved from http://www.jstor.org/stable/3583454

MoFPED. (1996). *Uganda Demographic an Health Survey 1995: Summary Report.* Entebbe, Uganda: Statistics Department: Ministry of Finance and Economic Planning.

MOH . (n.d.). *ADOLESCENT SEXUAL AND REPRODUCTIVE HEALTH IN UGANDA; Results of the AYA BASELINE SURVEY.* Kampala: Ministry of Health. Retrieved from library.health.go.ug/download/file/fid/180

MOH. (1999). *Uganda National Health Policy.* Kampala: Ministry of Health.

MOH. (2001). *The National Policy Guidelines and Service Standards for Reproductive Health Services: Reproductive Health Division; Community Health Department.* Kampala: Ministry of health.

MOH. (2010). *HEALTH SECTOR STRATEGIC & INVESTMENT PLAN.* Kampala: Ministry of Health.

MOH. (2012). *UGANDA AIDS INDICATOR SURVEY 2011.* Kampala and Calverton Maryland: Ministry of Health and ICF International.

Musoke, R. (2014, February 18). *Ugandan women needlessly dying from unsafe abortion.* Retrieved from THE INDEPENDENT: www.independent.co.ug/news/news/8720-ugandan-women-needlessly-dying-from-unsafe-abortion

Nalwadda, G., Mirembe, F., Byamugisha, J., & Faxelid, E. (2010). Persistent high fertility in Uganda: young people recount obstacles and enabling factors to use of contraceptives. *BMC Public Health.* Retrieved from http://www.biomedcentral.com/1471-2458/10/530

Nalwadda, G., Mirembe, F., Tumwesigye, N. M., Byamugisha, J., & Faxelid, E. (2011). Constraints and prospects for contraceptive service provision to young people in Uganda: providers' perspectives. *BMC Health Services Research.*

Nansubuga , R. (2011). Factors Affecting the Utilization of Antenatal Care Services among Adolescent Pregnant Mothers: Case Study of Naguru Teenage Health Center, Kampala, Uganda. *Int.statistical Inst.*

Neema , S., Musisi, N., & Kibombo, R. (2004). *Adolescent Sexual and Reproductive Health in Uganda: A Synthesis of Research Evidence.* New York & Washington: The Alan Guttmacher Institute.

Population Policy data Bank. (n.d.). *Uganda Abortion Policy.* Retrieved from Population Division: Department of Economic and Social Affairs of the UN Secretariat: www.un.org/esa/population/publications/abortion/doc/uganda.doc

population Secretariat, & UNFPA. (2012). *The State of Uganda Population Report 2012: Uganda at 50 years: Population and Service Delivery; Challenges, Opportunities and Prospects.* Kampala: Population Secretariat Ministry of Finance, Planning and Economic Development (MOFPED) .

PRB. (2009). *The World Population Data Sheet 2009.* Washington DC.: Population Reference Bureau.

Rosen, J. E. (2005, September). *USAID.* Retrieved from Youth Reproductive Health Policy Country Brief Series No.5; Uganda: Networking for Policy Change: http://www.policyproject.com/pubs/YRHCBS/Uganda%20country%20brief.pdf

Rutaremwa, G. (2013). Factors Associated with Adolescent Pregnancy and Fertility in Uganda: Analysis of the 2011 Demographic and Health Survey Data. *Social Sciences, 2*(1), 7-13.

Ssengooba, F., Neema, S., Mbonye, A., Sentumbwe , O., & Onama, V. (2004). *Health Systems Development Programme: Maternal Health Review Uganda.* Kampala: Makerere University Institute of Public health.

UBOS. (2008). *Population Dynamics Analytical Report.* Kampala: Uganda Bureau of Statistics.

UBOS, & ICF International. (2012). *Uganda Demographic and Health Survey 2011 .* Kampala and Maryland: UBOS and Calverton, .

UBOS, & Macro International Inc. (2007). *Uganda Demographic and Health Survey 2006.* Calverton, Maryland: Ubos and Macro International Inc.

UBOS, & UNFPA. (2014). *National Population and Housing Census 2014; Provisional Results.* Kampala: Uganda Bureau of Statistics .

Uganda Aids Commission. (2014). *THE HIV AND AIDS UGANDA COUNTRY PROGRESS REPORT 2013.* Kampala: Uganda Aids Commission.

Uganda Aids Commission. (2015). *THE HIV AND AIDS UGANDA COUNTRY PROGRESS REPORT 2014.* Kampala: Uganda Aids Commission.

Wallace, A. (2011, November). *Adolescent pregnancy and Policy Responses in Uganda.* Retrieved from Africa Portal: dspace.africaportal.org/jspui/bitstream/123456789/35416/1/backgrounder%2014.pdf?1

WHO. (2011, Nov 30). *The Partnership for Maternal, Newborn and Child Health.* Retrieved from Maternal And Child Health: Uganda: www.who.int/pmnch/media/membernews/2011/ugandabackgroundpaper.pdf

WHO. (2014, May). *Country Operation Strategy at a Glance.* Retrieved from World Health Organisation: http://www.who.int/countryfocus/cooperation_strategy/ccsbrief_uga_en.pdf

World Bank. (2015). *Data; Maternal Mortality Ratio.* Retrieved from The World Bank: data.worldbank.org/indicator/SH.STA.MMRT

World Bank. (2016). *Adolescent fertility rate (births per 1,000 women ages 15-19) .* Retrieved from The World Bank (Data): http://data.worldbank.org/indicator/SP.ADO.TFRT/countries

Worldwatch , I. (2016, March 22). *Uganda on Track to Have World's Highest Population Growth.* Retrieved from Worldwatch Institute: www.worldwatch.org/node/4525

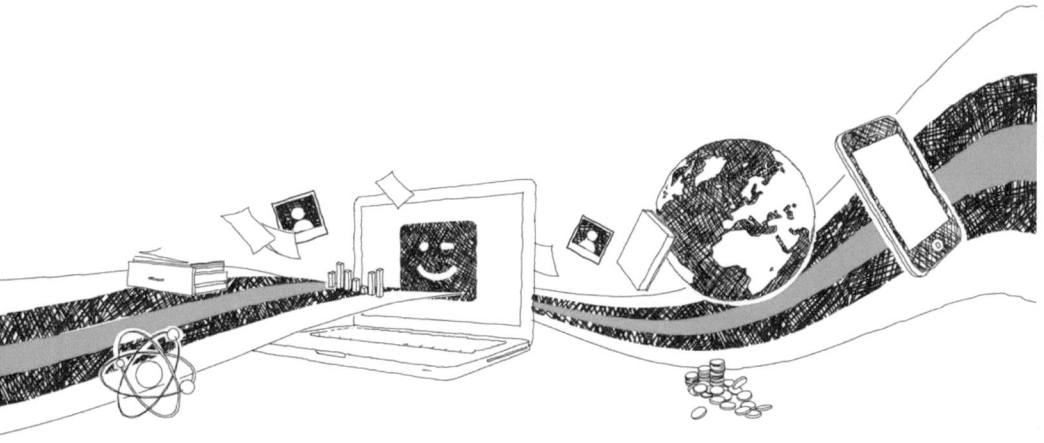
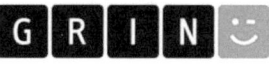